The Way of the Cross
for Caregivers to the Sick

Br. Ronald (Ted) Tokarz, O.F.M.

A Liturgical Press Book

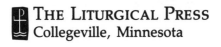

THE LITURGICAL PRESS
Collegeville, Minnesota

Cover design by Fred Petters.

I wish to acknowledge two people who planted the seed for this work, watered it with their support, and edited the manuscript: Mary Suciu and Sandy Reap.

Introduction

Lord, I wish to walk the Way of the Cross with you. I wish to make this my personal Way of the Cross, for I have a need to unburden my feelings, my fears, my anxieties, and above all to speak of my needs and the needs of those for whom I care. I am overwhelmed by the pain and suffering that surrounds me. There are times when I am depressed and even indifferent. I need support, I need an occasional hug but most of all, I need your strength to continue caring for those who are unable to take care of themselves. Help me to find those hidden sources of strength and a sense of fulfillment in the service of those who need me.

I

Jesus Is Condemned to Death

Leader: Lord, I stand before you totally drained. Caring for the sick, the aged, the abused, the terminally ill, the emergency cases can so deplete my energies and leave me emotionally, physically and psychologically drained. Even my spiritual resources seem to have deserted me. I need the support of others and above all, I need yours, O Lord.

Leader: Lord, source and fountain of strength,
People: **be our support, comfort and strength as we care for others.**

All: **Lord, there are times when we become weary and tired. We feel drained and no longer the powerhouses of energy that we thought ourselves to be. We are called upon to treat our patients with tender, loving care, but it is sometimes so difficult. We feel so dried up and giving becomes hard. Help us, Lord, especially at such times when caring becomes "just another job" rather than a labor of love. We ask this in the name of the loving and caring Lord, Jesus.**

II
Jesus Takes Up His Cross

Leader: Lord, I get up each day knowing that it will be a long and demanding one. The cross that I bear is not so much that of physical pain and suffering, as that of emotional care and concern for those who are suffering. Dispose my heart to the cries of those who are hurting. Give me an ear that willingly listens and a mouth that responds with words of comfort.

Leader: Lord, source and fountain of strength,
People: **be our support, comfort and strength as we care for others.**

All: **Lord, each day brings with it fears and anxieties which all contribute to our feelings of exhaustion. We move from one room of pain and suffering to another. We realize how fortunate we are and we thank you, but at the same time, we ask that you help us show compassion to those we care for. They have need not only of our hands and feet, but also our hearts and soothing touch. We ask this in the name of the loving and caring Lord, Jesus.**

III
Jesus Falls the First Time

Leader: Lord, there was a time when I saw myself as an "angel of mercy." I thought I had a bottomless source of energy whereby I could change the meaning of pain and suffering. But, I slowly began to realize that I too am human and can easily become tired, grouchy, and have bad days. Lord, help me to get up and continue doing, not so much great things, as things that make life more bearable for those I care for.

Leader: Lord, source and fountain of strength,
People: **be our support, comfort and strength as we care for others.**

All: **Lord, there are times when our caring for others becomes mechanical and artificial. We become preoccupied with many things in our personal lives, and lose sight of and feeling for the pain and suffering around us. Let the care and concern we have for others touch and alleviate the pain and suffering of those we care for. We ask this in the name of the loving and caring Lord, Jesus.**

IV
Jesus Meets His Loving Mother

Leader: Lord, I come into contact daily with many people who are in need of my assistance. For some, it is hard to lose independence and control. They look at me more with fear than suspicion which may cause them to become belligerent and even, incorrigible. They are afraid of what is happening and will happen to them. Help me, Lord, to allay their fears and anxieties by kindness, understanding and compassion.

Leader: Lord, source and fountain of strength,
People: **be our support, comfort and strength as we care for others.**

All: **Lord, we all have the mother in us. Upon meeting your mother, you must have felt the sorrow, love and compassion that emanated from her person. Those we care for seek our comfort, support and compassion and we can't fail them. They are our mothers and our fathers, our brothers and our sisters, yes, even our children. Compassion and care makes no distinction, they are not selective. Help us to care lovingly for all those in our care. We ask this in the name of the loving and caring Lord, Jesus.**

V

Simon Helps Jesus Carry His Cross

Leader: There are times when I feel so alone, so weighed down by the pain and suffering with which I come into contact daily. These feelings of helplessness and depletion are sometimes conveyed to my patients. At such times, I need your help in carrying out my work of caring. I need to seek the support of my peers lest my personal disposition interfere with the care I owe my patients. Help me, Lord, don't allow me to become ineffective.

Leader: Lord, source and fountain of strength,
People: **be our support, comfort and strength as we care for others.**

All: **Lord, sometimes it takes a long time before we come to the realization that we can't do everything alone. We need others and we especially need you to make up for all that is wanting in ourselves. We too need support and understanding, an occasional hug or a pat on the back. We too have needs that must be cared for. We need a helping hand, a friendly smile and an attentive ear that can help to reinforce our commitment to caring for others. We ask this in the name of the loving and caring Lord, Jesus.**

✝

VI

Veronica Wipes the Face of Jesus

Leader: In the process of caring for others, I have the opportunity to wipe away fluids and ease the hurts and pain. Your image is reflected in these people in spite of the many disfigurements their bodies bear. You have taken the form of suffering humanity. When I minister to them, I minister to you. Help me, Lord, to see you in them. Imbue me with that tender, loving care that so characterized you, my Jesus.

Leader: Lord, source and fountain of strength,
People: **be our support, comfort and strength as we care for others.**

All: **Lord, you told us that whoever shows a kindness to others, shows it to you. We perform many works of kindness for those who need our care: washing away the blood and body fluids and performing various ministrations for the body. Help us to treat the sick and the aged as if they were you. May our hands be gentle and our hearts compassionate. We ask this in the name of the loving and caring Lord, Jesus.**

✝

VII
Jesus Falls a Second Time

Leader: Lord, there are so many pitfalls in my work of caring for others. My humanness, with all that it entails, sometimes gets in the way of caring for my patients. I may be physically tired, emotionally drained, psychologically upset which tend to make me impatient and edgy. Help me, Lord, to catch myself at such times and don't let these feelings interfere with relieving the pain and suffering of those I care for.

Leader: Lord, source and fountain of strength,
People: **be our support, comfort and strength as we care for others.**

All: **Lord, we constantly come face to face with our shortcomings and humanness. Unfortunately, they can affect our dealings with those we care for because our moments of impatience and gruffness can add to the pain and suffering our patients already feel. Help us, Lord, to be conscious of moments of irritability lest they undo the good which we have already accomplished. Our patients need our personal attention and not our patronization. We ask this in the name of the loving and caring Lord, Jesus.**

VIII
Jesus Meets the Weeping Women

Leader: Lord, many are the times that my eyes fill with tears upon seeing the suffering and pain of those with whom I come into contact. These tears allow me to be sensitive to suffering humanity and are, at the same time, a source of compassionate helplessness that urges me to do what I can to alleviate their pain and suffering.

Leader: Lord, source and fountain of strength,
People: **be our support, comfort and strength as we care for others.**

All: **Lord, help us to be sensitive to the pain and suffering of others, and also to realize our limitations while doing so. Just as we seek support, an attentive ear and a hug, so do those to whom we minister. Let us act as if everything depended upon us, and pray as if everything depended upon God. We ask this in the name of the loving and caring Lord, Jesus.**

IX
Jesus Falls a Third Time

Leader: Lord, taking care of others day after day can cause me to become indifferent to them. I know that my work can even become monotonous and mechanical. Help me to realize that I am dealing with people who have feelings, needs and dreams. Some have lost their perception of reality, and others have lost their dreams. Hopes have disappeared and even died. I must try to be a source of strength to those I care for, reaffirming their faith and restoring their hope while ministering to their pains and suffering. Be my strength, Lord.

Leader: Lord, source and fountain of strength,
People: **be our support, comfort and strength as we care for others.**

All: **Lord, you are the source of all that is good, all that is holy. Help us to be a caring people who are able to reach out with faith and hope to those who are suffering. Help us to believe in your goodness and radiate it just as the rays of the sun dispense warmth and joy to a world that is in need of healing.**

X

Jesus Is Stripped of His Garments

Leader: Lord, there are many times when I feel stripped of all my energies, good will and good intentions. I don't have anything else to give. How easy it is to forget that it is in giving that I too receive. Even St. Paul tells me that I will find strength in my weakness. I come to you, Lord. I ask you to make up for all that is wanting in my response to those who need my care.

Leader: Lord, source and fountain of strength,
People: **be our support, comfort and strength as we care for others.**

All: **Lord, you remind us that in order to be your disciples, we must give up everything and follow you. At one time or another, each of us has had the opportunity to confront this truth. To lose or give up someone or something that is near and dear to us can be very traumatic. We need the assurance that you will always be there to comfort us, that you will turn the bitterness into sweetness and that the hundred-fold you promised us will not be denied us. We ask this in the name of the loving and caring Lord, Jesus.**

XI

Jesus Is Nailed to the Cross

Leader: Lord, I see so much pain and suffering. So many people are nailed to their beds of suffering. With tears in my eyes I try to relieve their distress. With eyes full of pain, bodies racked with fever and mutilated by disease, the sick, the aged, and the terminally ill turn to me for comfort and strength. They are helpless and I fear that they expect too much from me. Help me, Lord, to do what I can.

Leader: Lord, source and fountain of strength,
People: **be our support, comfort and strength as we care for others.**

All: **Lord, by asking us to bear our daily crosses, you also ask us to nail ourselves upon them. It isn't just our sins that we nail to our crosses, but also our sucesses and our failures, our accomplishments and our limitations, our joys and our sorrows, our needs and all that we have and are. Pain and suffering are part of the nailing process whereby the suffering of Christ is continued in our own bodies. With Christ, we continue his work of salvation. Help us, Lord, to be strong. We ask this in the name of the loving and caring Lord, Jesus.**

✝

XII

Jesus Dies Upon the Cross

Leader: Lord, so many have died that I once cared for. The young, the old, the sick, even the healthy—death does not discriminate. I feel so sad, so cheated when death steals another life from my care. But, I must never forget that death is not the end of life. Rather, it is the door which opens up to eternal life, the gateway that leads to eternal happiness. I will surely miss them, but I am content knowing that they will be eternally happy and free from pain and suffering.

Leader: Lord, source and fountain of strength,
People: **be our support, comfort and strength as we care for others.**

All: **Lord, we must all face death. We tend to forget that we are here on this earth as pilgrims and strangers journeying to our heavenly home. That place will be one of everlasting happiness where pain and suffering no longer exist, where tears will not be shed in sorrow and where true love, you, Jesus, will be our eternal light and joy. When that time comes, Lord, help us to direct our patients toward this goal with a faith and hope that will never waver: for it is in dying that we are born to eternal life. We ask this in the name of the loving and caring Lord, Jesus.**

✝

XIII
Jesus Is Taken Down from the Cross

Leader: Lord, how often I seek to be released from the stress? How often do I feel as if I am burning out, that I don't have anything more to give? How many times have I thought of going into another career? I stand back and look at my life. Where does one find freedom from pain and suffering? I have chosen to be a caretaker, and it disturbs me that when things get difficult I choose to flee, to give up. Help me, Lord, to do the best with what I've got, and not to accept defeat when things don't go right.

Leader: Lord, source and fountain of strength,
People: **be our support, comfort and strength as we care for others.**

All: **Lord, so often we come to the brink of burn-out, of indifference or of admitting defeat. We tire so easily allowing our emotions to override logic. We have need of you, not only at such times as this, but at all times. Help our minds to function clearly and our strength to be replenished. We need one another to talk to, to lean on, to comfort and support. We must utilize recreational outlets where our work is not the topic of conversation and where we are able to refresh our minds and bodies before resuming our ministry of caretaker. We ask this in the name of the loving and caring Lord, Jesus.**

✝

XIV

Jesus Is Laid in the Tomb

Leader: Lord, your bruised and torn body was finally laid to rest in a stranger's grave. How often I too seek rest when I am physically, emotionally and psychologically exhausted. How often I tire of seeing all these sick around me? How often I want to call it quits? But, in spite of this, I still return to my patients and begin all over again. I'm sure you, Lord, have a hand in this, and you sustain me, for it is your strength that carries me through my daily routine. It is your smile, your "thank you" that I see and hear on the lips of the suffering; it is your light that shines through those feverish eyes. I feel that I have much to give, but much more to receive.

Leader: Lord, source and fountain of strength,
People: **be our support, comfort and strength as we care for others.**

All: **Lord, you speak to us through the eyes, smiles and sufferings of the sick, the aged and the dying. You ask us to care for these, your children, as if it were you. Our dedication will not go unnoticed or unrewarded, for we willingly care for the members of your body. We are given a trust and are asked to do the best we can, nothing more is expected. We ask, Lord, in your name, that we may be the dispensers of your love and your care.**

✟

XV
The Resurrection

Leader: Lord all life is precious to you. Yet, you allow death to put an end to earthly life in order to raise us up to a life that is eternal. Our God has overcome death, he is the victor. He speaks to us through pain and suffering and assures us that all of this was not in vain. Their meaning may not be clear to us, but they are not only important, but also necessary. Help us, Lord, to place all our trust in you. May our faith and hope be renewed so that we may firmly believe that our ministry as caretakers is a positive contribution to this world. We are entrusted with the care of the sons and daughters of the Most High God. Because we bind up wounds, and ease pain and suffering in this world we can truly glory in the words of the Lord: eye has not seen, ear has not heard, nor has it entered into the mind of any one person, what great things God has prepared for those who love him. What better way can we show this love than by caring for the sick members of the People of God, the Church Suffering.